AF306962

Judith Gueswendé PITROIPA

LYMPHOMA OF THE LYMPH NODE MARGINAL ZONE

Judith Gueswendé PITROIPA

LYMPHOMA OF THE LYMPH NODE MARGINAL ZONE

LYMPHOMA OF THE GANGLION MARGINAL ZONE AT THE FADA N'GOURMA REGIONAL HOSPITAL (BURKINA FASO)

ScienciaScripts

Imprint

Any brand names and product names mentioned in this book are subject to trademark, brand or patent protection and are trademarks or registered trademarks of their respective holders. The use of brand names, product names, common names, trade names, product descriptions etc. even without a particular marking in this work is in no way to be construed to mean that such names may be regarded as unrestricted in respect of trademark and brand protection legislation and could thus be used by anyone.

Cover image: www.ingimage.com

This book is a translation from the original published under ISBN 978-620-6-72115-4.

Publisher:
Sciencia Scripts
is a trademark of
Dodo Books Indian Ocean Ltd. and OmniScriptum S.R.L publishing group

120 High Road, East Finchley, London, N2 9ED, United Kingdom
Str. Armeneasca 28/1, office 1, Chisinau MD-2012, Republic of Moldova, Europe
Printed at: see last page
ISBN: 978-620-8-10222-7

DEDICATIONS AND THANKS

To Almighty God.

Who inspired me, who guided me along the right path, I owe what I have become to you, submission, praise and thanks.

To Mum and Dad.

I dedicate my success to you today. May God, the merciful, welcome you to his eternal paradise, AMEN!

To my children : Hope Axel Johan and Ange Priscille Kiswendsida. You have made many sacrifices during your training. May this work of yours inspire you to always work hard and give the best of yourselves. May God bless you all.

To my brothers and sisters: Colette, Fréderic, Victorien, Emmanuel, Roland, Edwige and Basile Junior. Brotherhood is priceless, as they say. Thank you so much for being with me all these years. I will always need you for the rest of my career. Please accept the expression of my brotherly love! This work is a credit to you! May we remain united by the grace of God!

To my nephews: Ethan, Dylan Yanis and Maël, you are angels. May God bless you, grant you a long life and make you pious beings who are loved by HIM. I love you all.

ACKNOWLEDGEMENTS

Our thanks go to :

*To **Professor Assita SANOU/LAMIEN,** my teacher and dissertation supervisor. Thank you for your guidance and for the knowledge I have acquired at your side. May the Lord in his great goodness shower you with blessings.*
*To my co-supervisor, **Dr Souleymane OUATTARA**, dear master, thank you for agreeing to correct this work. I am at a loss for words to express my gratitude. May the Almighty repay you a hundredfold for all your kindnesses.*

To all the staff supervising the master's degree in clinical cytology at the UFR/SDS of Joseph KI-ZERBO University, thank you, dear masters, for all the rich practical teaching I have received. It was a real pleasure and honour for me to learn from you.

*To all the staff of the Pathological Anatomy and Cytology Department of the Fada N'Gourma Regional Hospital, especially my colleague and head of department, **Dr HIEN Téontoume**, thank you very much. May the Almighty keep us together, amen.*

TO OUR MASTERS AND JUDGES

To our Master and Chair of the Jury, **Professor Olga Mélanie LOMPO**
You are

⚜️***Full Professor of Anatomy and Pathological Cytology at the UFR/SDS
Joseph KI-ZERBO University;***

⚜️***Head of Department of Anatomy and Pathological Cytology, CHU Yalgado
Ouédraogo ;***
⚜️***Holder of the CHAIRE Recherche et Action Contre le Cancer (ReAAC);*** ⚜️
Head of the School's Morphology and Organogenesis Laboratory
Doctorale des Sciences et Santé (ED2S) at the Université Joseph KI-Zerbo; ⚜️
Coordinator of the Master in Clinical Cytology;
⚜️***Chevalier de l'Ordre National ;***

⚜️***Chevalier de l'Ordre International des Palmes Académiques (OIPA) of
CAMES.***

Honourable master,

*It is an immense privilege that you have given us by agreeing to chair this work.
In working with you over the last few years, dear Master, we have come to
appreciate your simplicity, your scientific rigour and your love of a job well
done. You taught us pathological anatomy and clinical cytology, and introduced
us to research, which was my first step into this essential discipline that you
cherish so much. We will be eternally grateful to you.*

Our dearest wish is to continue to benefit from your immense knowledge.

May Almighty GOD bless you abundantly!

To our Master and supervisor, **Professor Assita SANOU/ LAMIEN**

You are

Full Professor of Anatomy and Pathological Cytology at the UFR/SDS of Joseph Ki-ZERBO University;

Deputy Head of the Pathological Anatomy and Cytology Department at the Yalgado Ouédraogo University Hospital;

Coordinator Diploma specialised studies in Pathological Anatomy and Cytology;

Deputy coordinator of the Masters in Clinical Cytology ;

President of the Société Burkinabé de Pathologie (SOBUPATH); Director of the Ecole Doctorale des Sciences et Santé (ED2S);

Chevalier de l'ordre du mérite national agrafe santé; Chevalier de l'ordre de l'Etalon.

Honourable Master,

Your scientific knowledge, your simplicity, your friendliness, your scientific rigour and your love of a job well done are all admirable.

We have were very impressed by your accessibility, your availability at all times.

Please accept our sincere thanks.

May Almighty God accompany you throughout your life!

To our Master and Judge, **Professor Cheikh Bougadari TRAORE**

You are

⚜Professor of Pathological Anatomy and Cytology at the Faculty of Medicine and Odontostomatology (FMOS);

⚜Head of the Fundamental Sciences Teaching and Research Department at the FMOS of the University of Science, Technology and Technology of Bamako (USTT-B);

⚜Head of Department of Anatomy and Pathological Cytology at the Centre Hospitalier Universitaire (CHU) Point G ;

⚜Director of the Mali Cancer Registry ;

⚜Director of the Centre for Research and Training in Molecular Pathologies (CREFPAM);

⚜President of the Malian Pathology Society (SMP);

⚜Collaborator in the cervical cancer screening project in Mali.

Dear Master,

We are very grateful for the honour you have done us by agreeing to sit on our dissertation defence jury, despite your busy schedule. Please allow us to express our admiration for your spontaneity and kindness in agreeing to judge this modest work.

May God bless you and repay you for all the sacrifices you have made over the many years of your career. Amen.

TABLE OF CONTENTS

INTRODUCTION

Lymphomas are haematological malignancies that arise from the abnormal proliferation of mature lymphocytes of the B lineage in 85% of cases and of the T lineage in 15% of cases. B lymphomas account for the majority of cases and comprise a large number of heterogeneous entities, both in terms of clinical presentation and prognosis [1].

Lymphomas are subdivided into 2 categories: Hodgkin lymphomas and non-Hodgkin lymphomas (NHL). Non-Hodgkin's lymphoma is the ninth most common cancer, with more than 355 new cases diagnosed each year in Burkina Faso [2].

Classified as indolent B-type NHL, marginal zone lymphomas (MZL) account for 11% of all NHL [3]. The lymphocyte at the origin of these marginal zone lymphomas is a rather special cell known as a "memory" cell. It is a lymphocyte that has retained the memory of a previous interaction with a foreign agent (antigen) and is therefore capable of producing a rapid and highly adapted immune response. These memory B lymphocytes are stored in an area of the lymph nodes known as the "marginal zone". It is from this zone that the abnormal lymphocytes spread, hence the name of the disease. In the fifth edition of the World Health Organisation classification [4], marginal zone lymphomas include three entities: extraganglionic MZLs developed from mucosa-associated lymphoid tissue (MALT) found mainly (70%) in the stomach, splenic MZLs (SZMLs) (20 %) and lymph node MZL (LZMG) (10%) [5, 6]. What these entities have in common is a generally indolent course, with a limited risk of transformation into a high-grade lymphoma. While considerable progress has been made in understanding the pathophysiological mechanisms of MALT lymphoma, which is the paradigm of a tumour triggered by a chronic antigenic stimulus, there is still much to be done, LZMG is relatively rare. We report a case of LZMG in a 52-year-old man diagnosed in the pathological anatomy and cytology department of the Fada N'gourma Regional Hospital. There is very little data available on LZMG, which prompted this study, the aim of which was to identify the diagnostic approach based on the exclusion of other types of small B-cell NHL.

1. GENERAL

1.1 THE LYMPHATIC SYSTEM

1.1.1 ANATOMICAL REMINDER

The lymphatic system is part of the body's defence system. It is made up of :

- Lymph nodes: these are small bean-shaped organs found throughout the body.

- Lymphatic vessels: vessels that allow lymphatic fluid to circulate throughout the body.

- Other organs: bone marrow, thymus, tonsils, spleen, liver, lymphoid tissue associated with mucous membranes [7].

Figure 1 shows a diagram of the lymphatic system.

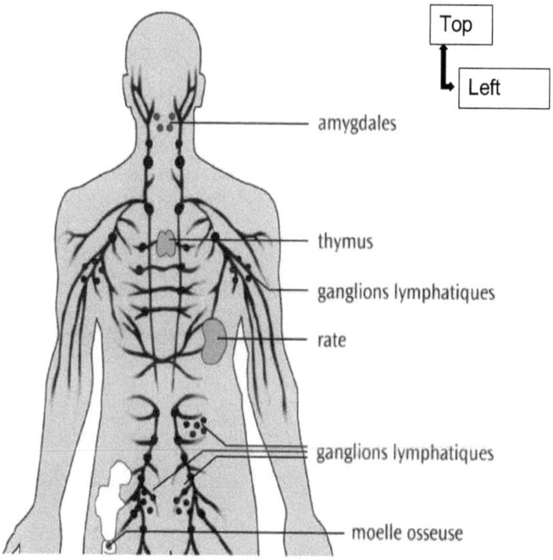

Figure 1: Diagram of the lymphatic system [7].

1.1.2 HISTOLOGY OF LYMPH NODE TISSUE

Lymph nodes are surrounded by a fibrous capsule and divided by trabeculae of connective tissue that arise from the capsule and meet at the hilum. They consist of a superficial cortex, a central medulla and a deep cortex (or paracortex) at the interface of the two [7] .

The superficial cortex is made up of lymphocytes mainly arranged in spherical lymphoid follicles; these are the main sites for the localisation and proliferation of B lymphocytes. Lymphoid follicles are classified as "primary follicles" if they do not have a clear centre, and as "secondary follicles" if they do. Primary follicles are essentially made up of B lymphocytes and are transformed into secondary follicles after antigenic stimulation. From the periphery towards the centre, these are made up of :

- Marginal zone: surrounding the mantle zone, not normally visible in lymph nodes. The marginal zone is a distinct anatomical compartment, composed of B cells, well developed in lymphoid organs subject to abundant antigenic influx, such as the spleen, Peyer's patches of the small intestine and tonsils. It is less obvious in lymph nodes, with the exception of mesenteric lymph nodes [7]. The marginal zone is part of the lymphoid follicle. It surrounds the ring of mantle lymphocytes and is composed of medium-sized lymphocytic elements, with a nucleus containing one or two nucleoli, and pale cytoplasm of varying abundance. It is associated with a few small lymphocytes, macrophages, polymorphs and plasma cells [7].
- The mantle zone: located at the periphery of the follicle, made up of small, naïve lymphocytes.

- Germinal centres: site of B lymphocyte proliferation, characterised by the presence of a dense and complex network of follicular dendritic cells, centroblasts and centrocytes, T lymphocytes and some macrophages.

- The medullary cords contain mainly B lymphocytes and plasma cells involved in the synthesis of immunoglobulins.

- The deep cortical zone, or paracortex, is essentially made up of T lymphocytes which are never grouped together in follicles [8].

Figure 2 shows a schematic cross-section of a lymph node.

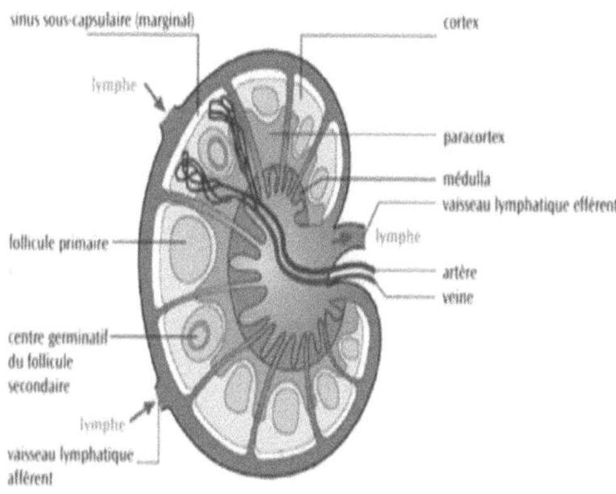

Figure 2: Structure of the lymph node [8].

Figure 3 shows the normal histological appearance of a lymph node at low magnification.

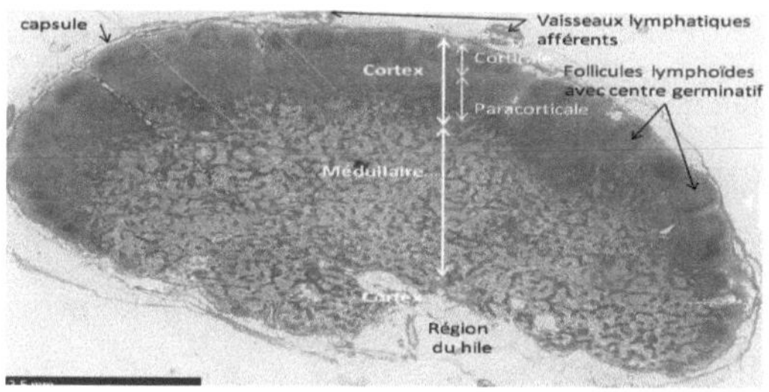

Figure 3: Normal histology of a lymph node (HE, G40) [8].

Figure 4 shows the normal histological appearance of a lymph node at intermediate magnification.

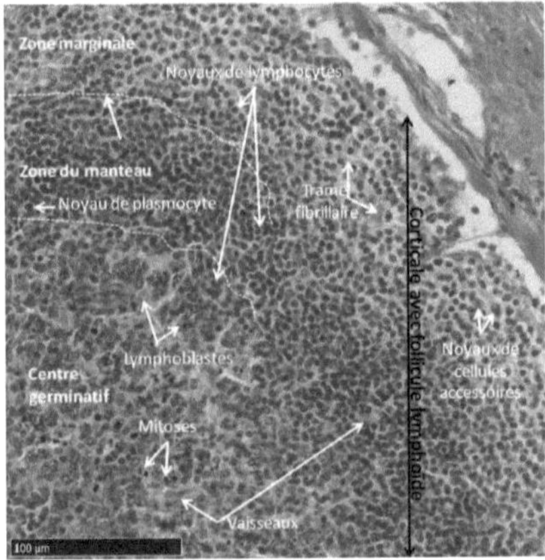

Figure 4: Normal histology of a lymph node at intermediate magnification (HE, G100), [8].

1.2 B LYMPHOCYTE DIFFERENTIATION

B lymphocytes mediate humoral immunity and immunological memory. To carry out these functions, these cells must undergo a number of differentiation steps enabling them to acquire the widest possible repertoire of antigen receptors (antibodies), which are nonetheless tolerant to self. Some of these stages, involving somatic remodelling of gene segments and refinement of their specificity (through a process of somatic hypermutation), are complex and, although highly regulated, not without danger for the integrity of the genome. The first stages in the development of B lymphocytes take place in the bone marrow, and allow assembly of the antigen receptor through the process of recombination [9]. In adults, B cells, at this stage still The "immature" B lymphocytes leave the bone marrow and reach the spleen, where a fundamental cellular decision will direct their destiny towards either a T-independent (TI) or a T-dependent (TD) response [10]. This decision depends on the type of signalling involved, to which each transitional B lymphocyte is differentially sensitive. This first developmental bifurcation will give rise on the one hand to pre-activated marginal zone B cells residing in the splenic marginal zone, and on the other hand to mature follicular B cells residing in splenic follicles. In humans, the origin of marginal zone B cells is still debated, and these lymphocytes may not originate from this lineage of transitional cells, but rather from the liver or possibly from mucosa-associated lymphoid tissue (MALT) [11]. These marginal zone B cells are specifically educated to respond rapidly to blood-borne IT antigens, and produce a first line of defence of the It is an "innate" protection against specific pathogens such as encapsulated bacteria. In humans, most (if not all) marginal zone B lymphocytes carry levels (albeit relatively low) of somatic hypermutations on the variable regions of their receptors, suggesting that receptor diversification may occur outside the classical TD response, and prior to antigen encounter.

The development of B lymphocytes is shown in Figure 5.

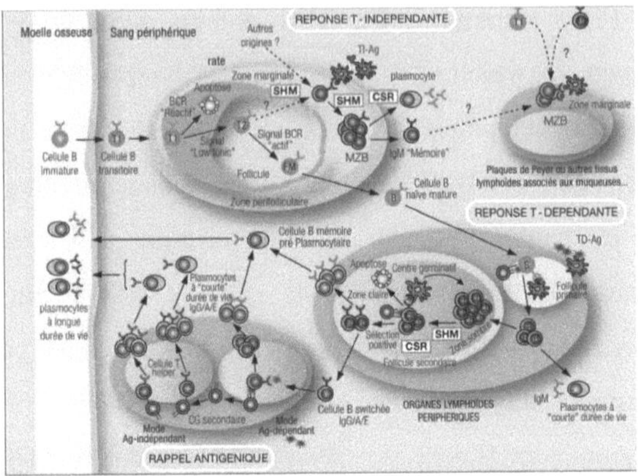

Figure 5: Diagram of B lymphocyte development [11].

Legend: SHM: somatic hypermutation; CSR: class switching; TI-Ag: T-independent antigen; TD-Ag: T-dependent antigen; MZB: marginal zone B lymphocytes; cc: centrocyte; cb: centroblast. Upon antigenic stimulation, pre-activated, pre-diversified and pre-developed marginal zone B lymphocytes rapidly migrate into the bloodstream either as antibody-secreting plasma cells or as IgM memory B lymphocytes.

In contrast, mature follicular B lymphocytes are not yet effector cells when they leave the spleen and recirculate in the bloodstream. These naïve B cells have not yet encountered their specific antigen, but they are primed to respond functionally to TD stimulation. This latter reaction occurs in the follicles of the secondary lymphoid organs. When naive B lymphocytes enter the peripheral lymphoid organs, they are directed towards a primary follicle, which they scan for the presence of an antigen. These B lymphocytes, now activated by the antigen, rapidly relocate to the B-T inter-follicular zone, where they undergo an initial limited expansion under the impetus of the signal, resulting from interaction with T cells (via the T receptor and the CD40/CD40L pair in particular). A fraction of the cells differentiate into short-lived IgM plasma cells, which undergo neither class switching nor somatic hypermutation, but rapidly produce an initial response to invasive pathogens. The other fraction of activated B cells initiates the formation of a germinal centre (GC) in a secondary follicle. In the dark zone of the germinal centre, the activated B cells repress surface expression of the antigen receptor, as well as other genes such as Bcl2, proliferate extensively as centroblasts, and trigger the affinity maturation programme, consisting mainly of the process of somatic hypermutation of immunoglobulin genes. As the process of somatic hypermutation is random, mutations in the antigen receptor will in most cases result in a reduction in affinity for the antigen by which these cells were initially stimulated, and only a small minority will be assigned a more affine receptor. The centroblast-centrocyte transition is accompanied by cell cycle arrest, migration into the light zone of the GC, and a second crucial decision for the cell. The mutated receptor is re-expressed on the cell surface and "tested" by helper follicular T cells (hFTCs) and presenter dendritic cells (DCs) [12]. Depending on the new affinity of its receptor for the antigen, the centrocyte is either ignored and dies by apoptosis (when affinity is decreased); or instructed to restart a cycle of mutations (when affinity is unchanged); or instructed to undertake class switching and complete the final stages of CG maturation (when affinity is increased). Hypermutated, switched and differentiated follicular B cells re-express a certain number of genes such as Bcl2 and exit the GC for a fraction as switched memory B lymphocytes expressing IgG, IgA or IgE of high affinity for the antigen, and for another fraction having undergone massive expansion and terminal differentiation as short-lived plasma cells secreting IgG, IgA or IgE isotype antibodies. A fraction of these plasma cells recirculate in specific niches in the bone marrow and acquire a longer lifespan (a few months). Switched memory B lymphocytes recirculate to peripheral lymphoid organs (in particular back to the spleen), where they become the key regulators of the long-term memory response to recurrent infectious episodes. During these infectious recalls, two modes of response take place:

- In the classic "antigen-dependent" mode, switched antigen-specific memory B cells are reactivated via their receptor by the corresponding helper T cells and undergo a new cycle of massive clonal expansion and differentiation into plasma cells;

- In a recently proposed "antigen-independent" mode, polyclonal stimulation of the pool of switched memory B cells resident in the secondary lymphoid organs where antigen recall takes place is simultaneously stimulated collaterally by an indirect aid, antigen-independent T cell proliferation (so-called bystander effect, possibly via CD40-CD40L interaction and cytokine production). This effect is thought to lead to (more limited) proliferation of memory B cells with non-specificities to the invading pathogen, and differentiation into a new generation of plasma cells [13].

These recurrent polyclonal activations of the global pool of memory B cells during successive antigenic challenges in an individual's immunological history could explain the long-term production of a broad spectrum of antibodies, and therefore the maintenance of a serological memory throughout human life.

1.3 CLASSIFICATION OF B LYMPHOMAS

In 2008, the World Health Organisation (WHO) classification of haematological malignancies established the existence of three entities depending on the site of involvement: MZL, MZSL and MZLG. This classification was expanded in 2016 to include monoclonal B lymphocytosis of the LZM type and red pulp lymphoma or other borderline forms [4].

The B lymphomas in the 2016 WHO classification are grouped together in TableI.

Table I: WHO 2016 classification of B lymphomas [4].

Mature B lymphoid neoplasia
Chronic lymphocytic leukaemia / Lymphocytic lymphoma
Monoclonal B lymphocytosis *
Prolymphocytic B leukaemia
Splenic marginal zone lymphoma
Hairy cell leukaemia
Splenic B lymphoma/leukaemia, unclassifiable
Diffuse small-cell B lymphoma of the splenic red pulp
Hairy cell leukaemia - variant
Lymphoplasmacytic lymphoma
Waldenström's macroglobulinemia
Monoclonal gammopathy of undetermined significance (MGUS) IgM *
Heavy chain disease m
Heavy chain disease g
Heavy chain disease a
Monoclonal gammopathy of undetermined significance (IgG/IgA*)
Multiple myeloma
Solitary plasmacytoma of bone
Extraosseous plasmacytoma
Monoclonal Immunoglobulin Deposition Disease * (MID)
Extra-ganglionic marginal zone lymphoma of mucosa-associated lymphoid tissue (MALT)
Ganglion marginal zone lymphoma
Pediatric lymph node marginal zone lymphoma
Follicular lymphoma
Follicular neoplasia in situ
Duodenal-type follicular lymphoma *
Paediatric follicular lymphoma* (PFL)
Large B-cell lymphoma with IRF4 * rearrangement
Primary cutaneous centrofollicular lymphoma
Mantle cell lymphoma
Mantle cell neoplasia in situ * (MCN)
Diffuse large B-cell lymphoma (DLBCL), without other specificity (NOS)
type B of the Germinal Centre *
type Activated B *
Large B-cell lymphoma, rich in T lymphocytes/histiocytes

Primary DLBCL of the central nervous system
Primary cutaneous DLBCL, leg type
DLBCL EBV+, NOS *
EBV+* mucocutaneous ulcer
DLBCL associated with chronic inflammation
Lymphomatoid granulomatosis
Primary mediastinal (thymic) large B-cell lymphoma
Intravascular large B-cell lymphoma
ALK+ large B-cell lymphoma
Plasmablastic lymphoma
Serous lymphoma
DLBCL HHV8+, with no other specificity*.
Burkitt's lymphoma
Burkitt-like lymphoma with 11q aberration *
High-grade B lymphoma, with rearrangement of MYC and BCL2 and/or BCL6 *
High-grade B lymphoma, NOS
Unclassifiable B lymphoma, with intermediate features between DLBCL and classic Hodgkin's lymphoma

1.4 MARGINAL ZONE LYMPHOMAS

1.4.1 DEFINITION

MZLs represent a group of lymphomas in which the cells are derived from B lymphocytes normally present in the marginal zone (MZ) of secondary lymphoid follicles [14]. These cells are anatomically localised in lymphoid organs (spleen and lymph nodes) and non-lymphoid organs that can be separated into mucosal lymphoid tissue [MALT] and non-mucosal lymphoid tissue such as the skin, orbit or dura mater. They were included as a provisional entity in the revised European and American classifications [15], then as a separate entity in the World Health Organisation classification [4]. The International Lymphoma Study Group has identified 3 distinct subgroups of marginal zone lymphomas, depending on their sites of invasion [15] :

- LZME or MALT lymphoma,

- LZMS (with or without lymphocytes),

- LZMG (with or without monocytoid cells).

These lymphomas may present in a disseminated form from the outset. Histological transformation into a large cell lymphoma may occur at diagnosis or during the clinical course. Despite this classification, the relative rarity of these lymphomas and the difficulties in distinguishing them from other low-grade lymphomas, especially when they are disseminated, are obstacles to carrying out accurate epidemiological analyses and describing their clinical course.

Figure 6 shows the three entities of marginal zone lymphoma.

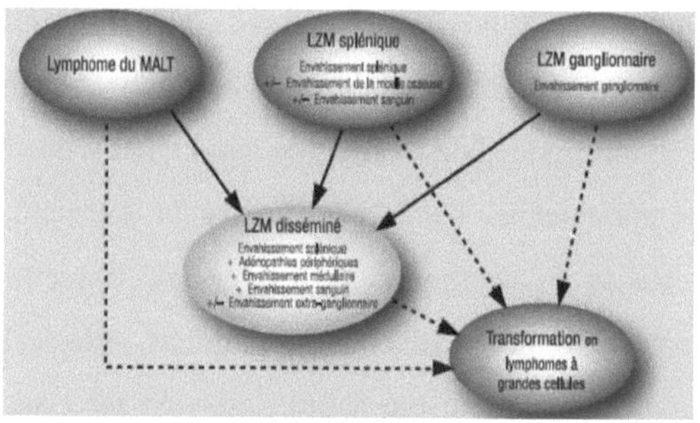

Figure 6: The three entities of marginal zone lymphoma [15].

1.4.2 POST-GERMINATIVE ORIGIN OF MARGINAL ZONE LYMPHOMA

The origin of NHL of the marginal zone is therefore a memory B lymphocyte of the marginal zone and, by definition, of post-germinative origin, as shown by the study of somatic mutations in the genes for the variable part of the heavy chains (VH) of immunoglobulins. However, it has recently been shown that these lymphomas have a heterogeneous mutational profile, with one third of cases having a non-mutated profile and two thirds a mutated profile [17]. Furthermore, these lymphomas show a low frequency of somatic mutations in certain oncogenes (Bcl6, PAX5, PIM1, RHO-H). This confirms that the cellular origin of LZMs is distinct from the B cells of GCs and suggests that the cells of origin may not have passed through the GC [17].

1.4.3 ROLE OF RECEIVER B AND CHRONIC ANTIGENIC STIMULATION

The survival and selection of B lymphocytes depend on their BCR, even in the mature and quiescent stage. This survival signal is delivered autonomously or secondary to antigen activation (pre-BCR). In the case of NHL, the BCR signal is also necessary for survival, as demonstrated by the absence of BCR-negative variants in lymphomas and the fact that the B receptor in lymphoma cells continues to undergo somatic hypermutation. There is increasing evidence that MALT, splenic or lymph node MZLs may be associated with chronic antigenic stimulation, either endogenous by autoantibodies or exogenous by microbial pathogens. This leads to an accumulation of lymphoid tissue in typical sites of invasion of this lymphoma in the mucous membranes, spleen, lymph nodes, or in organs not normally containing lymphoid tissue. In the case of autoimmune stimulation, several diseases have been associated with the risk of developing MALT lymphoma, such as Hashimoto's thyroiditis, sialic myoepithelial adenitis with or without Gougerot Sjogren's syndrome, or lymphoid interstitial lung disease. Based on epidemiological studies, molecular investigations and effective therapeutic approaches, five microbial pathogens have now been identified as being linked to marginal zone lymphoma. Helicobacter pylori is the best characterised and has been associated with gastric MALT lymphoma [18]. The best described infections to date are hepatitis C virus infection and Helicobacter pylori infection. In the case of LZMS with more or less villeous lymphocytes, a clear link with HCV has been demonstrated [19]. The HCV E2 glycoprotein is thought to interact with CD81 of the B lymphocyte, and to be responsible for B lymphocyte activation via BCR signalling, thus contributing to their lymphomagenesis. The reduction in lymphoproliferation with antiviral treatment supports the role of this chronic antigenic stimulation in the pathophysiology of HCV-associated MZL [20].

Figure 7 illustrates marginal zone lymphomas associated with chronic antigenic stimulation.

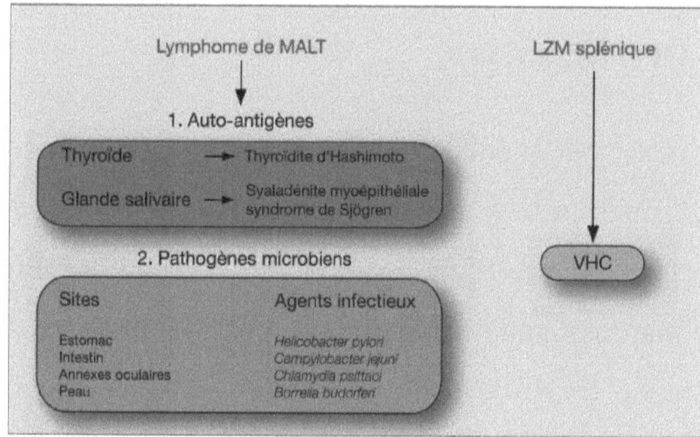

Figure 7: Marginal zone lymphomas associated with chronic antigenic stimulation [20].

1.5 LYMPHOMA OF THE LYMPH NODE MARGINAL ZONE (LZMG)

MGL is a small-cell NHL that originates in the lymph node, with a histological and immunohistochemical appearance resembling a lymph node site of MALT-type MGL or MSSL, with no evidence of a primary lymphoma outside the lymph node or spleen [4].

1.5.1 EPIDEMIOLOGY OF LZMG

LZMG is a relatively rare indolent lymphoma, accounting for 1-2% of all lymphoid neoplasms and approximately 10% of all LZMs [4, 21]. The median age at diagnosis is 55-60 years [4, 21]. The incidence of LZMG is similar in men and women [4, 21]. It can also be diagnosed in children where it has distinct clinical and morphological features with excellent prognosis [4, 22]. In the 2016 WHO classification of tumours of haematological and lymphoid tissues, 'paediatric LZMG' is described as a distinct variant [4].

1.5.2 HISTORY OF THE LZMG

Initially called lymph node monocytoid B lymphoma by Sheibani et al. in 1986 [26], Cousar et al. referred to it as parafollicular lymphoma in 1987 because of the morphological appearance of the infiltration [27]. In 1988, Piris et al. made the link with the marginal zone compartment [28], which led to its inclusion in the Kiel classification in 1990. The 2001 WHO classification presents it as a provisional entity [29], then in 2008, the same classification definitively identifies it as one of the three MZLs [30]. This is the least well described LZM.

1.5.3 CLINICAL AND PARACLINICAL ASPECTS OF LZMG

The majority of patients present with disseminated disease involving peripheral (frequently inguinal and cervical) and deep (most often abdominal and thoracic) lymph nodes. Although spinal cord involvement is less common than in MSSL, it is most commonly described in half of cases, with variations ranging from 15 to 62% of cases [31, 32]. Clinical signs such as asthenia, fever, weight loss and anorexia are rare. Biologically, cytopenias are rare. Elevation of $\beta 2$ microglobulin occurs in a third of patients. The presence of cryoglobulin is associated with HCV infection. Unlike other marginal zone lymphomas and apart from autoimmune haemolytic anaemia, no autoimmune manifestations have been described in this lymphoma [33].

1.5.4 ANATOMOPATHOLOGICAL DIAGNOSTIC METHODS

➤ Cytological study

In the event of clinical suspicion of lymph node lymphoma, cytological sampling by fine needle aspiration of an adenopathy is carried out to detect lymphoma. If the cytology is favourable to the diagnosis, it is followed by a histological study with immunohistochemistry to confirm the lymphoma and specify its characteristics [5, 6].

➤ Histopathological study

Diagnosis can be made by transcutaneous needle biopsy. This type of sampling is preferred for lymphomas that are difficult to access [8]. For superficial lymphadenopathies or lymphadenopathies accessible to surgery, complete lymph node excision is preferable [8]. Whenever possible, it is preferable to remove the largest lymph node, outside the axillary, inguinal or retro crural lymph nodes, which are often reorganised [34]. The sample should be sent intact as soon as possible.

➤ Immunohistochemical study

IHC plays a vital role in the diagnosis and appropriate classification of lymphomas. It may also have prognostic value [3, 8]. This technique is used to search for the expression of surface or intracellular antigens using labelled antibodies directed against these antigens [35].

➢ **Cytogenetic and molecular methods**

Classical cytogenetics, which analyses the morphological appearance of chromosomes in metaphase cells, is currently supplemented by molecular biology techniques, which are playing an increasingly important role in the diagnosis of lymph node lymphoma. The two main techniques used are FISH and PCR [29, 35].

1.6   ASPECTS MORPHOLOGICAL, CYTOGENETIC AND MOLECULAR ASPECTS OF LZMG

1.6.1 MORPHOLOGICAL ASPECTS OF LZMG

Histologically, LZMG shows great architectural and cytological variability. At low magnification, multiple architectural patterns can be observed. Lymphocyte proliferation may be diffuse, interfollicular, perifollicular or nodular. Signs of colonisation of germinal centres can be misleading, particularly in cases which have been diagnosed as large cell lymphoma [4, 36, 37]. In some cases, a A "splenic" follicle with centrifugal growth from the marginal zone of follicles with reduced mantle and residual GCs. At higher magnification, LZMG cells show a heterogeneous morphology, ranging from centrocyte-like cells to monocytoid cells to plasmacytoid cells, with variable numbers of centroblasts and immunoblasts interspersed. Monocytoid cells have a central nucleus with condensed chromatin and indistinct nucleoli, surrounded by pale clear cytoplasm. The cells, which sometimes resemble the centrocytes of the germinal centre, have nuclei with slightly irregular nuclear membranes and a coarser chromatin structure. Lymphoplasmacytic cells are visible and have some of the characteristics of plasma cells. They are smaller than typical plasma cells with less basophilic cytoplasm and have a finer chromatin structure. In the rare cases where monocytoid cells predominate, secondary involvement of the lymph nodes by a MALT-type lymphoma should be considered. A floral variant has also been reported. This variant is characterised by a proliferation of medium-sized cells in the marginal zone surrounding enlarged GCs, with a thick, irregular mantle zone that sometimes extended into the GC, similar to progressively transformed GCs.Infiltration of the bone marrow has only been described in a small number of cases, with nodular and paratrabecular architecture in most cases, rarely diffuse. The impact of the percentage of large cells on prognosis and the dividing line between diffuse large B-cell lymphoma and DLBCL remain unclear. Some authors have diagnosed transformation if more than 20% of large cells are visible. However, this phenomenon is fairly rare.[38, 39, 40].

Figure 8 illustrates the histological aspect of the diffuse architecture of lymphoma of the lymph node marginal zone.

Lymphocytic proliferation of diffuse architecture with effacement of lymph node architecture.

Figure 8: Marginal zone lymphoma of diffuse architecture (HE, G40) [38].

Figure 9 illustrates the histological appearance of follicular lymph node marginal zone lymphoma.

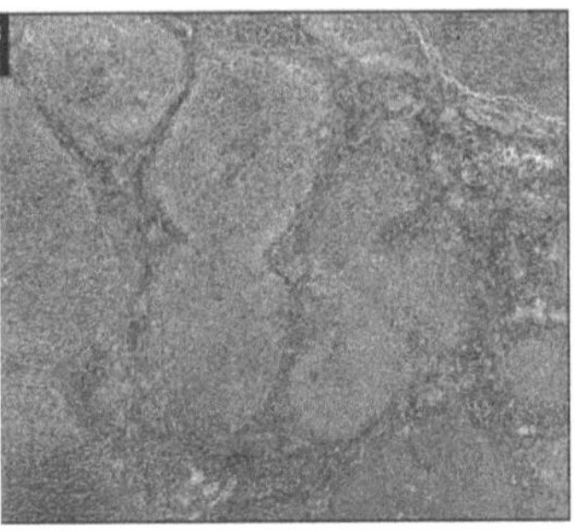

Proli arhitrcture nodular/follicular characterised by well-defined distinct, well-demarcated nodules with areas inter follicular not

Figure 9: Follicular marginal zone lymphoma (HE, G40) [38].

Figure 10 illustrates the histological aspect of lymphoma of the ganglion marginal zone of perifollicular architecture.

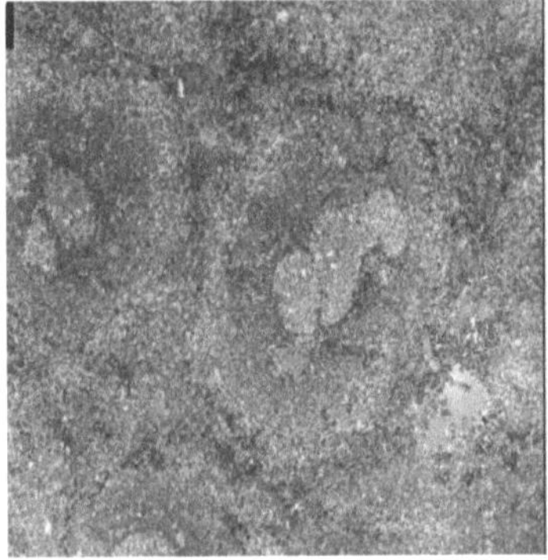

Proliferation lymphocytic perifollicular, characterised by an annular distribution of tumour lymphocytes around normal secondary follicles not infiltrated by lymphoma cells.

Figure 10: Lymphoma of the perifollicular marginal zone (HE, G40) [38].

Figure 11 shows the histological appearance of lymph node marginal zone lymphoma with a plasmacytoid appearance.

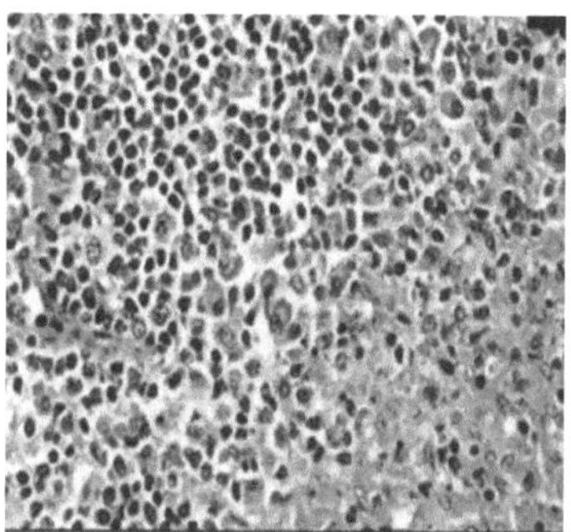

Cells tumos scattered plasma cells, abundant cytoplasm abundant eosinophilic, often nucleolated.and figures some mitotic. clarified Presence

Figure 11: Marginal zone lymphoma with a plasmacytoid appearance (HE, G100) [38].

The histological appearance of lymph node marginal zone lymphoma with a monocytoid appearance is shown in Figure 12.

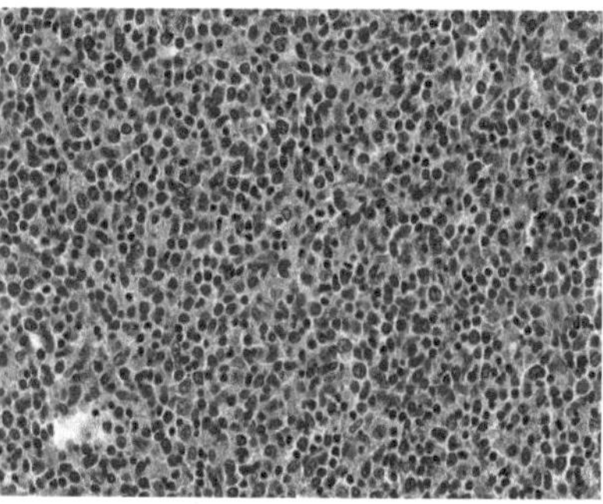

Lymphocyte proliferation consisting of small tumour lymphocytes with cytoplasms basophilic and with irregular hyperchromatic nuclei.

Figure 12: Marginal zone lymphoma with monocytoid appearance (HE,200) [40].

Figure 13 shows the histological appearance of lymph node marginal zone lymphoma at high magnification.

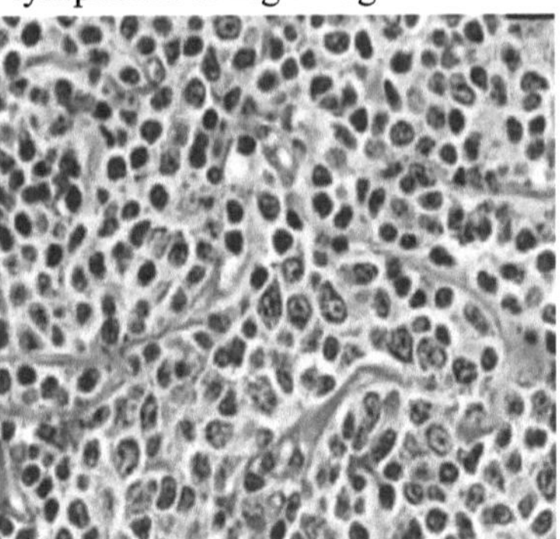

Small to medium-sized lymphomatous cells with sparse, eosinophilic cytoplasm, (eosinophilic monocytoid), nucleolated nuclei, sparse, sclerotic stroma

Figure 13: Lymphoma of the lymph node marginal zone observed at high magnification (HE, G400) [38].

Figure 14 shows lymphoma of the lymph node marginal zone at high magnification.

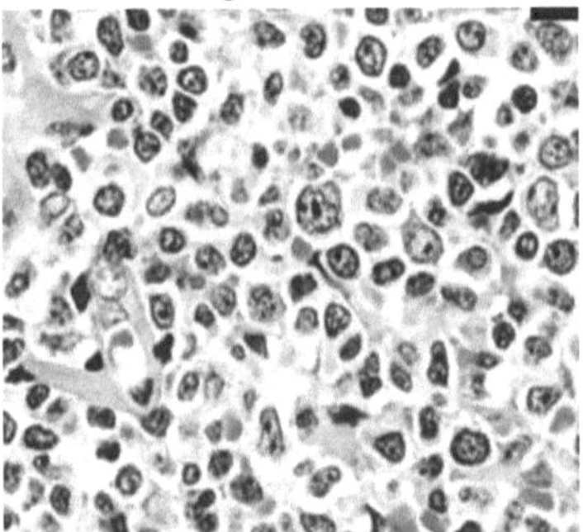

Medium to large tumour cells with moderately abundant moderately abundant cytoplasm, irregular nuclei with often condensed, often fine dusty chromatin and nucleolated

Figure 14: Lymphoma of the lymph node marginal zone observed at high magnification (HE, G400) [38].

1.6.2 IMMUNOHISTOCHEMICAL ASPECTS OF LZMG

There is no specific marker for this lymphoma, so its diagnosis is one of elimination and requires rigorous integration of clinical, morphological, immunohistochemical and molecular elements. Tumour cells express pan-lymphocytic B markers: CD20, CD79a, Oct2, BOB1 and PAX5, although CD20 expression may be reduced in cases of strong plasma cell differentiation. Tumour cells also express Bcl2 and CD43 in 20-75% of cases. In the case of plasma cell differentiation, plasma cells are positive for MUM1 markers. In paediatric LZMG:CD20, CD43 and Bcl2 markers are positive in 50% of cases [38, 39, 40].

The figure 15 shows microscopic of LZMG after immunostaining with anti-CD20.

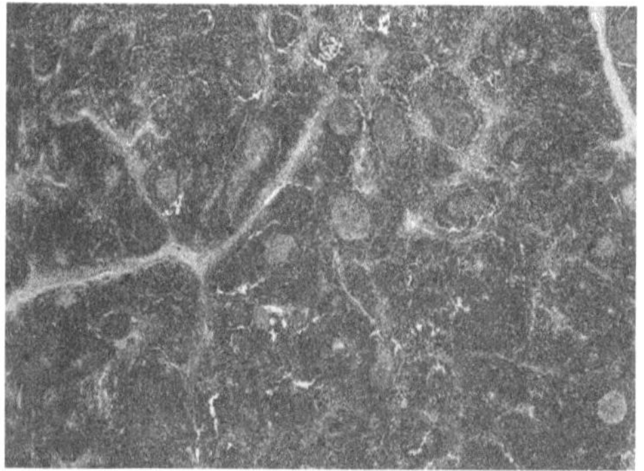

Marking intense cytoplasmic and diffus from cells lymphomatous by anti-CD20 Ac.

Figure 15: Immunostaining of LZMG with anti-CD20 Ac, G40 [40].

The figure 16 shows microscopic of LZMG after immunostaining for Bcl2.

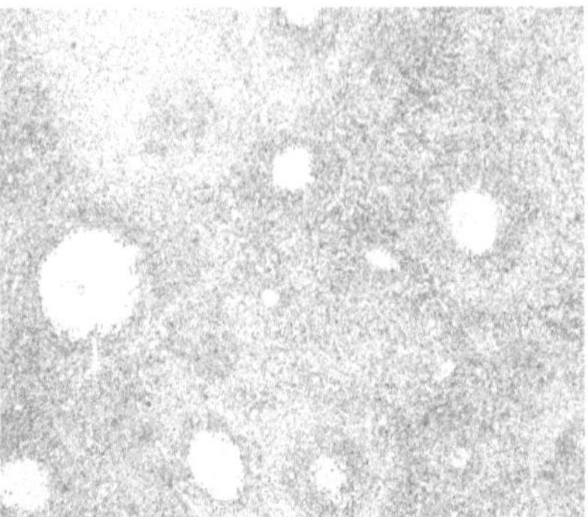

Diffuse and intense cytoplasmic labelling of lymphoma cells by anti-Bcl2 Ac. The germinal centres are negative.

Figure 16: Immunostaining of LZMG with anti-Bcl2 Ac, G40 [40].

Figure 17 shows the microscopic appearance of LZMG after PAX5 immunostaining.

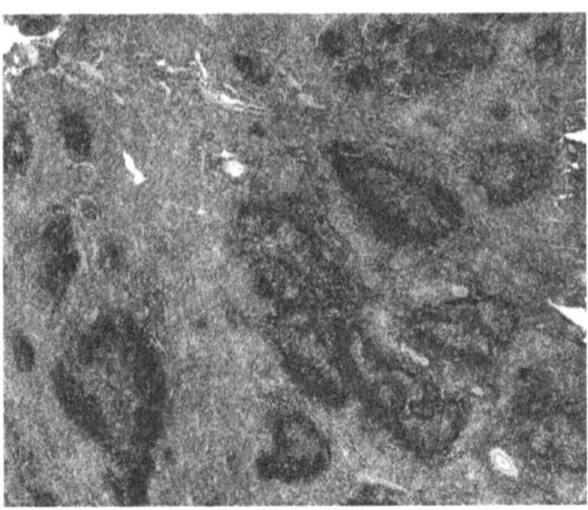

Nuclear expression of PAX5 by follicular and inters follicular tumour cells.

Figure 17: Immunolabelling of LZMG with PAX5, G40 [40].

1.6.3 CYTOGENETIC AND MOLECULAR DATA ON LZMG

In terms of cytogenetics, numerous chromosomal abnormalities have been identified. These can be detected by conventional karyotyping after tumour cell culture or by chromosomal analysis using a DNA microarray (ACPA) after DNA extraction. Chromosome gains of 1q, 2p, 3p, 3q, 6p and 6q are frequently reported [6]. Loss of chromosomes 1q and 6q, as well as trisomies 3, 12 and 18 have been described. Monosomies 9, 13 and 14 are rarer. However, these anomalies are not specific to LZMG [41]. In LZMG, mutations were observed in the NFκB signalling pathway including CARD11 (~7%), MYD88 (5-13%), and IKBKB (~7%) and in that of TNFAIP3 (A20) (7-13%), BIRC3 (API2) (~6%) and TRAF3 (~5%). These mutations are mutually exclusive. The L265P mutation in the MYD88 gene is reported in a small proportion of cases (6-9%). While mutations in NOTCH 2 and KLF2 are more specific to LZMS, mutations in TNFAIP3 and TRAF3 are more common in LZMG [42, 43].

1.7 LZMG EXTENSION ASSESSMENT

The extension work-up to be carried out for splenic and lymph node MZL is identical to that recommended for malignant lymphomas of other organs, with the following investigations:

- a thoracic-abdominal-pelvic CT scan, with a PET scan optional,

- a haemogram, myelogram and bone marrow biopsy,
- a biological work-up including LDH levels,

- serologies for hepatitis B, C and HIV,

- an autoimmunity test to look for rheumatoid factor and cryoglobulin, especially if hepatitis C serology is positive [43].

1.8 THERAPEUTIC STRATEGIES

The treatment of LZM is not standardised. There are few series in the literature
on the treatment of LZMG. The guidelines proposed here for patients seen in the
primary care setting are based on the most recent publications. Monitoring alone
appears to be the appropriate course of action for asymptomatic patients with a
small tumour mass.

1.8.1 TREATMENT OF LOCALISED LZMG

As with follicular lymphoma, patients with localised forms can be cured with 24
Gy of radiotherapy.

1.8.2 TREATMENT OF DISSEMINATED LZMG

• Asymptomatic patients who do not present any criteria for a tumour syndrome,
as defined by the GELF, are regularly monitored without treatment.
• Symptomatic patients with no tumour syndrome benefit from chlorambucil-
based monochemotherapy, ideally combined with rituximab [44].
• Patients with one of these criteria should benefit from rituximab-based
immunochemotherapy, such as "R-CVP" (rituximab, cyclophosphamide,
vincristine and prednisone), possibly combined with an anthracycline ("R-
CHOP") if there are poor prognostic factors. Bendamustine, in combination with
rituximab, is a very interesting drug in this indication [45, 46].
• Immunotherapy helps to strengthen or restore the immune system's ability to
fight cancer. Interferon-alpha may be given alone or in combination with a drug
called ribavirin, which is used to treat viral infections such as HCV [47, 48].

Figure 18 shows the treatment regimen for LZMG.

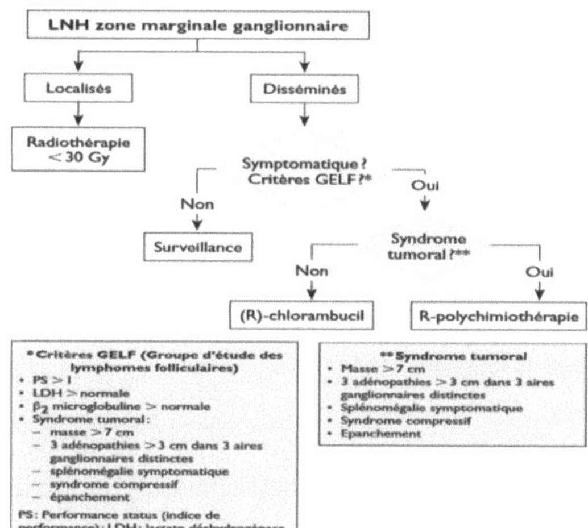

Figure 18: LZMG treatment regimen [51].

1.9 EVOLUTION, PROGNOSTIC FACTORS AND FOLLOW-UP

The outcome of these patients with LZMG is identical to that of patients with LZMS. Estimated 5-year survival for these patients is between 50 and 70% [51]. The course of NHL is divided into four stages known as Ann Arbor staging: stages I and II are localised, while stages III and IV are considered extensive or disseminated.

The characteristics of each stage are given in Table II [51].

Table II: Ann Arbor staging of NHL [51].

I IE	1 seul groupe ganglionnaire IE : 1 seul territoire extra ganglionnaire de contiguïté
II IIE	Plusieurs groupes ganglionnaires du même côté du diaphragme IIE : II + 1 territoire extra ganglionnaire de contiguïté
III	Plusieurs groupes ganglionnaires des 2 côtés du diaphragme
IV	Atteinte viscérale

Tumour mass is assessed according to the criteria of the GELF (Follicular Lymphoma Study Group), which has validated the following criteria [51] :

- A tumour mass > 7 cm.

- The presence of 3 adenopathies larger than 3 cm.

- The existence of general symptoms.

- Elevated serum levels of LDH or ß2-microglobulin.

- The presence of splenomegaly.

- The presence of compression or effusion.

Among the prognostic factors cited in the literature [52] are age over 60, an abnormal LDH level and poor general condition. As in the case of patients with MALT-type MZL, after treatment, patients are monitored clinically and biologically on a quarterly basis for two years, then semi-annually for three years and then annually. Imaging tests are only prescribed for patients with symptoms or clinical signs suggestive of progression.

1.10 DIFFERENTIAL DIAGNOSIS OF LZMG

Several diagnoses need to be discussed: all small cell lymphomas, but more particularly follicular lymphoma and mantle cell lymphoma, and above all lymphoplasmacytic lymphoma, with which there are borderline areas [37]. Confusion with lymphoplasmacytic lymphoma has no negative consequences for management.

2 OUR STUDY

2.1 OBJECTIVES

2.1.1 GENERAL OBJECTIVE

To study the morphological and immunohistochemical aspects of lymphomas of the lymph node marginal zone, based on a case encountered in the pathological anatomy and cytology department of the Fada N'Gourma regional hospital.

2.1.2 SPECIFIC OBJECTIVES

1- Study the clinical and paraclinical diagnostic approach to lymph node marginal zone lymphoma.

2- Study the histological and immunohistochemical diagnostic approach to lymph node marginal zone lymphoma.

3- To establish the therapeutic strategy for lymph node marginal zone lymphoma.

2.2 CASE OBSERVATION

52-year-old patient with chronic viral hepatitis B since 2018 on Tenofovir 300mg tablet whose last HBV viral load in August 2023 was undetectable. The symptoms began 9 months ago (May 2023) with the appearance of a left laterocervical mass with little pain. As the mass progressively increased and the pain intensified, the patient consulted the internal medicine department of the Fada N'Gourma Regional Hospital in October 2023 where he was already being treated for HBV infection. On admission, the patient was in good general condition with a WHO performance index of grade 1, with normal vital signs (systolic blood pressure 130mmHg, diastolic 80mmHg, pulse 104 beats per minute, temperature 36.7°Celsius). Examination of the cervical region revealed left laterocervical adenopathy. These adenopathies were superficial, firm, painful, non-pulsatile to palpation and mobile in relation to the deep and superficial planes; the skin opposite was healthy. The patient was given a prescription for painkillers and anti-inflammatory drugs, and an assessment of the adenopathies was carried out. The blood tests included a lactic dehydrogenase (LDH) test, which came back above normal (391.3 IU/L), and a Beta-2-microglobulin test, which also came back above normal (2.92mg/L). A cervico-thoraco-abdomino-pelvic CT scan with contrast injection revealed four (04) left latero-cervical adenomegalia measuring 18mm, 15mm, 14mm and 9mm; solid intra-abdominal and pelvic organs with no abnormalities; no fluid effusion; and no mediastinal, supra-clavicular or intra-abdominal adenomegalia.

Figure 19 shows a cervical CT scan of our patient.

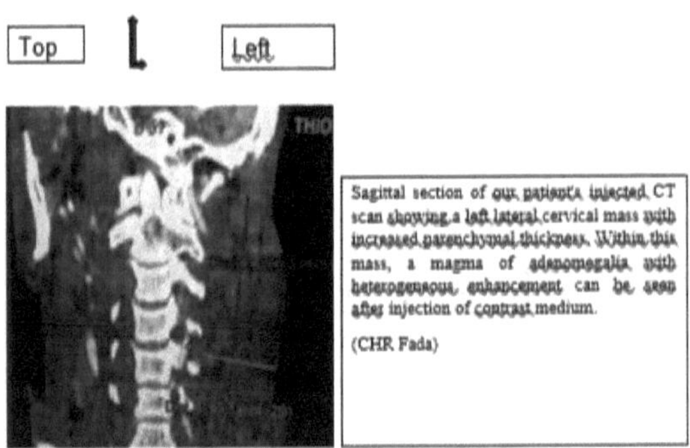

Sagittal section of our patient's injected CT scan showing a left lateral cervical mass with increased parenchymal thickness. Within this mass, a magma of adenomegalia with heterogeneous enhancement can be seen after injection of contrast medium.

(CHR Fada)

Figure 19: Cervical CT scan, sagittal section.

Faced with this diagnostic difficulty, the patient was referred to the general surgery department, where the pathological lymph nodes were removed. The specimen was sent to the pathological anatomy and cytology department of the Fada N'Gourma regional hospital where, after histological examination coupled with immunohistochemistry, a definite diagnosis of lymphoma of the lymph node marginal zone was made.

2.3 ANATOMOPATHOLOGICAL EXAMINATION

2.3.1 STUDY METHOD

The specimen was immediately immersed in 10% buffered formalin in the operating theatre before being transported to the laboratory. The container was large enough and the volume of formalin was sufficient - at least 10% of the volume of the specimen. This fixation allowed morphological conservation of tissue and cell structures. The sample was accompanied by a completed examination application form. At the laboratory, the sample was recorded and an appointment was made for a fortnight to collect the pathology result. Fragments were measured during macroscopy. The fragments were not oriented; they were described in their various aspects and a total inclusion was carried out. The specimen was then subjected to a so-called circulation stage, corresponding to dehydration, thinning and paraffin impregnation of the tissues. Inclusion consisted of making a paraffin block by orienting the fragment appropriately in the direction of the section. The paraffin block was cut to a thickness of 4 micrometres using a microtome. This thickness allows the microscope's light rays to pass through the sample and avoids cell superimposition. The sections were spread out on a slide and then stained using the standard technique that combines a nuclear stain (haematein) and a cytoplasmic stain (eosin), commonly known as H.E.Microscopic examination was carried out after mounting the preparation on a slide glued with a special glue called Eukit (this enables the slides to be preserved at a later date by preventing oxidation of the dyes and destruction of the tissue spreads).

The patient underwent an immunohistochemical examination: this is a method of locating proteins in the cells of a tissue section, by detecting antigens using antibodies. The revelation system was based on the enzymatic reaction between peroxidase, coupled to the dextran polymer, and the chromogen diaminobenzine (DAB) (Dako). The revelation system was based on the enzymatic reaction between peroxidase, coupled to the dextran polymer, and the chromogen diaminobenzine (DAB) (Dako). The markers used were CD20, Bcl2, CD5, CD10, CD23, Bcl1 and Ki67. The expected results were positive labelling for antibodies to CD20, Bcl2 and Ki67 and no labelling for antibodies to CD5, CD23, CD10 and Bcl1.

2.3.2 MACROSCOPIC EXAMINATION

Four (04) fragments weighing a total of 4 grams were received in 10% buffered formalin. The largest fragment was 12 mm long, 8 mm wide and 5 mm thick. The smallest fragment measured 7 mm in long axis. They were fibrous in appearance, blackish in colour, and had a firm elastic consistency. On sectioning, the fragments showed no remodelling.

2.3.3 MICROSCOPIC EXAMINATION

➢ **Standard histology**

After macroscopic examination, the sample was circulated using the usual technique. The paraffin block obtained was roughened and cut with a microtome to obtain thin ribbons which were spread out on a slide. The standard manual staining combining a nuclear dye (haematein) and a cytoplasmic dye (eosin) called HE was carried out. After this stage, microscopic examination revealed a tumour proliferation of diffuse architecture, completely obliterating the normal architecture of the lymph node. The tumour lymphocytes were small, with sparse eosinophilic cytoplasm. The nuclei are irregular, hyperchromatic, often clarified with a small nucleolus. Nuclear atypia were marked. Mitotic figures were rare and no necrosis was observed.

Figure 20 shows the histological appearance of the LZMG at low magnification.

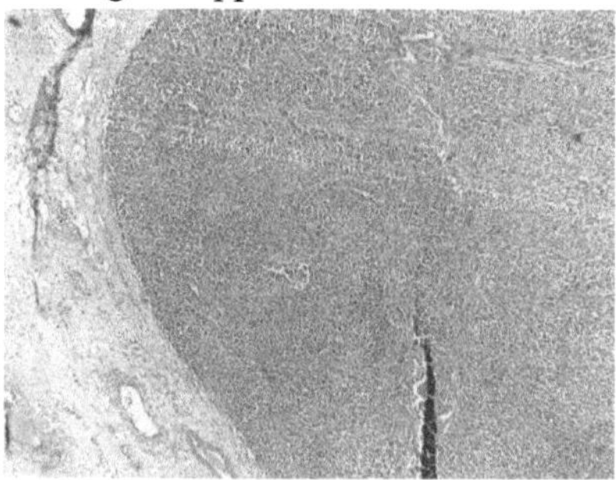

We observes a proliferation of diffuse diffused architecture erasing the normal

Figure 20: Lymphoma of the lymph node marginal zone (HE, G40) (Anatomy and pathological cytology laboratory of the Fada Regional Hospital Centre).

Figure 21 shows the histological appearance of the LZMG at intermediate magnification.

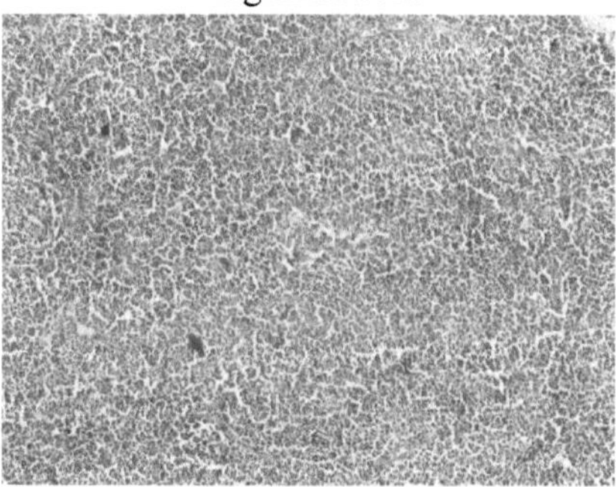

Lymphocytic cells tumour from small size

Figure 21: Lymphoma of the lymph node marginal zone (HE, G100) (Anatomy and pathological cytology laboratory of the Fada Regional Hospital Centre).

Figure 22 shows the histological appearance of the LZMG at high magnification.

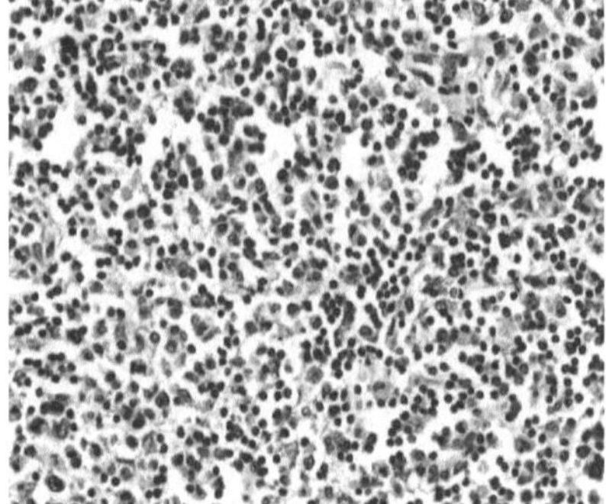

Small lymphomatous cells with sparse cytoplasm and irregular nuclei, hyperchromatic, clarified   ofeten a small with nucleoli.

Figure 22: Lymphoma of the lymph node marginal zone (HE, G400) (Anatomy and pathological cytology laboratory of the Fada Regional Hospital Centre).

> **Immunohistochemistry**

Afterwards, immunohistochemical labelling was carried out in the morphology and organogenesis laboratory of the doctoral school of science and health at the Joseph KI-ZERBO University in Ouagadougou.

This marking is obtained using a manual technique which works as follows:

- Dewax and rehydrate tissue sections on slides;

- Wash with distilled water for 1 minute, then 1 x 2 minutes;

- Unmask pressure cooker at 98°C (PH: 6 or 8) for 10 minutes;

- Remove the slides and allow them to cool to room temperature (RT) for about 45 minutes;

- Rinse for 1 minute then 1 x 2 minutes;

- Block endogenous peroxidases with the "Peroxide Block for image Analysis (ADA)" kit for 10-15 minutes;

- Wash with PBS buffer (diluted to)1X1 min then 1X2 min ;

- Neutralise the non-specific background noise (BDF) "Super Block ref (AAA)" in "Kit Ultra Tek HRP Anti polyvalent Lab Pak 12 ref: UHP125"5mn,

NB: do not exceed 10 minutes;

- Rinse with PBS buffer for 1 x 1 min, then 1 x 2 min;

- Apply the primary antibody (Ac) to the slides (Ac: dilutions chosen by reference to the supplier) for 30 minutes;

- Rinse with PBS buffer 1 x 1 min then 1 x 5 min;

- Amplify primary Ac with " Ultra Tek Anti-Polyvalent (ABN) " Kit " Ultra Tek HRP Anti polyvalent Lab Pak 12 ref : UHP125 "10mn ;

- Rinse with PBS buffer 1 x 1 min then 1 x 2 min;

- Apply "Ultra Tek HRP (ABL)" (primary Ac is localized by a universal secondary Ac (poly and monoclonal Ac) conjugated to a polymer labelled with 1 enzyme, Kit "Ultra Tek HRP Anti polyvalent Lab Pak 12 ref: UHP125" 10mm;

- Rinse with PBS buffer 1 x 1 min then 1 x 2 min and distilled water 1 x 1 min;

- Reveal the Ag/Ac complex with Diaminobenzydine (DAB) " Quanto Chromogen ref : TA 060QHDX " DAB Quanto Sustrat 1ml + 1 drop DAB (protect from light) 5mn ;

- Rinse with distilled water for 1 minute;

- Apply DAB a second time for 5 minutes;

- Rinse with PBS buffer 1 x 1 min then 1 x 2 min;

- Counterstain with haematoxylin for 1 minute;

- Rinse with distilled water for 1 minute, then 1 x 2 minutes;

- Immerse the slides in xylene ;

- Mount between slide and coverslip (EUKITT) ;

We obtained the following results for :

CD20: intense and diffuse positive labelling of the cytoplasm of tumour cells.

Bcl2: medium intensity, diffuse labelling of the cytoplasm and nuclear membrane affecting around 50% of tumour cells.

CD5: absence of tumour cell labelling.

CD3: no labelling of tumour cells.

Bcl1 or Cyclin D1: no labelling of tumour cells.

CD10: no labelling of tumour cells.

CD23: no labelling of tumour cells.

Ki67: high-intensity nuclear marking affecting around 30% of tumour cells.

The CD19, CD43, CD79a and PAX5 markers also requested were not immunostained because they were not available.

Figure 23 shows the microscopic appearance of LZMG after immunostaining with anti-CD20 Ac.

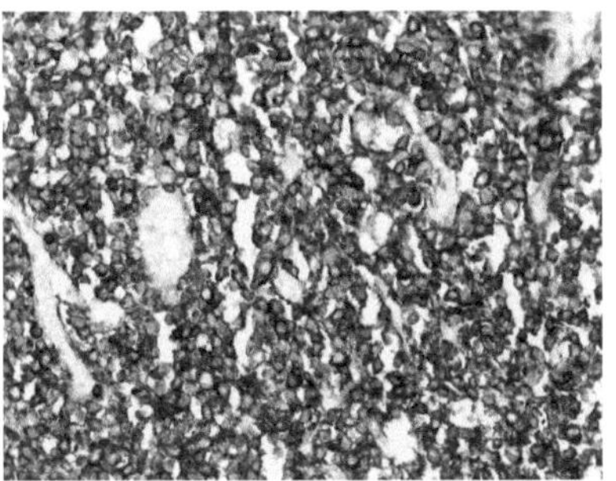

Marking membrane tumour cells to the anti-CD20 Ac.

Figure 23: Immunostaining of LZMG with anti-CD20 Ac, G400 (Morphology and organogenesis laboratory of the doctoral school of science and health at the Joseph KI-ZERBO University, Ouagadougou).

Figure 24 shows the microscopic appearance of LZMG after immunostaining for Bcl2.

Moderate and diffuse cytoplasmic and nuclear Bcl2 labelling by almost 50% of tumour cells.

Figure 24: Immunolabelling of LZMG with Bcl2, G40 (Morphology and organogenesis laboratory, doctoral school of science and health, Joseph KI-ZERBO University, Ouagadougou).

Figure 25 shows the microscopic appearance of LZMG after immunostaining with Ki67.

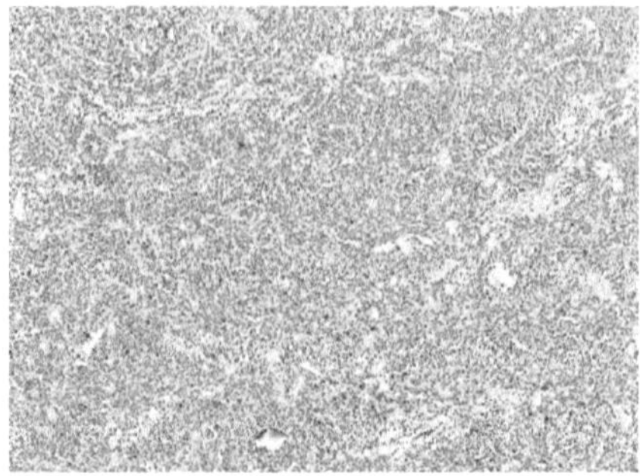

Figure 25: Immunolabelling of LZMG with Ki67, G40: intense nuclear labelling affecting approximately 30% of tumour cells. (Morphology and organogenesis laboratory of the doctoral school of science and health at the Joseph KI-ZERBO University in Ouagadougou).

This anatomopathological procedure led to the conclusion of lymphoma of the lymph node marginal zone. The patient was admitted for chemotherapy and the outcome was favourable, with a reduction in the left laterocervical mass and complete disappearance of the pain.

3. COMMENTS

Ganglion marginal zone lymphoma is a rare type of B-cell non-Hodgkin's lymphoma (NHL) that progresses slowly (indolent). The median age at diagnosis is between 55 and 60 years, with no gender predominance [4, 21, 41]. We report the case of a 51-year-old adult male. In studies by Mohamed Salama [38] and Sung Yong [53], on a cohort of 51 and 36 patients respectively, with ages ranging from 13 to 78 and 14 to 65 years, the median age at diagnosis was 55 and 60 years. Some studies have deduced that LZMG although common in adults, can also be diagnosed in children where it has distinct clinical and morphological features with an excellent prognosis [23, 24]. In the 2016 WHO classification of tumours of haematological and lymphoid tissues, "paediatric LZMG" is described as a distinct variant [4].

Histologically, paediatric LZMG presents morphological and immunophenotypic features comparable to adult LZMG. However, it is distinguished by its excellent prognosis and certain features such as infiltration of hyperplastic lymphoid follicles by lymphomatous cells, which take on the appearance of follicles undergoing progressive transformation. In children, there is a male predominance and most cases are asymptomatic with localised disease (stage I), a low relapse rate and an excellent outcome [23, 24].

In the vast majority of cases, the precise origin of non-Hodgkin's lymphoma remains unknown. It is generally accepted that the onset of non-Hodgkin's lymphoma is most often linked to a combination of behavioural, environmental and genetic risk factors. Like all cancers, non-Hodgkin's lymphomas are not contagious diseases. LZMG appears to develop on a background of chronic inflammation, sometimes linked to an infection (hepatitis B or C, HIV and, to a lesser extent, Epstein-Barr virus or cytomegalovirus) or an autoimmune disease (systemic lupus erythematosus, Sjögren's disease, rheumatoid arthritis). However, there is too little evidence to establish a causal link [32, 43, 49]. In our case, the patient had a history of viral hepatitis B. In our case, the LZMG was discovered in the form of a painful swelling on the left postero-cervical side, progressing slowly and gradually increasing in size. The patient's general condition was preserved and vital signs were normal. LZMG mainly affects the peripheral lymph nodes, and often presents as isolated asymptomatic peripheral adenopathy or polyadenopathy with preferential involvement of the lymph nodes of the head and neck.

The cervical region is the most commonly affected site. Extra-ganglionic extension at diagnosis is possible, with spinal cord involvement described in a third of cases [41]. From a biological point of view, blood tests carried out in the presence of adenopathy which may indicate lymphopathy are Beta-2-microglobulin, which is a first-line marker in multiple myeloma and malignant B lymphopathy, and the enzyme LDH (lactic dehydrogenase). These assays are of great interest in clinical biology as a tumour marker and index of progression and prognosis in various diseases of the haematopoietic system. They were abnormally high in our patient.The topographical diagnosis is made on the basis of imaging data, in particular CT scans, which show the location, number and size of pathological lymph nodes, and any locoregional extension. In our case, CT revealed four left lateral cervical adenomegalia measuring 18 mm, 15 mm, 14 mm and 9 mm. Any lymph node larger than 10 mm in diameter is considered pathological [54].

These pathological lymph nodes were located without involvement of other lymph node territories, or extra-local or distant lymph nodes. Whatever the organ involved, these lymphomatous lesions will present a certain number of common characteristics on imaging, which should lead to the diagnosis being evoked or the most frequent diagnoses of primary or secondary tumours being called into question, in order to encourage biopsy sampling [54].

In our case, the diagnosis was confirmed by pathological examination. The diagnosis can only be made with certainty by histology and IHC. Excisional biopsy of one or more lymph nodes is the preferred method. The integration of clinical, paraclinical, morphological, immunophenotypical and genetic data is essential for the diagnosis of lymphoma pathology. To date, there are no immunohistochemical or molecular markers specific to LZMG. As this is an uncommon disease, there are few series in the literature.Histologically, LZMG shows great architectural and cytological variability.

This architecture is diffuse in 75% of cases [38], sometimes with vague nodularity, in which case other small-cell B non-Hodgkin's lymphomas with a diffuse architecture should be ruled out. Cytological polymorphism is present in all series [37, 39, 42]. Monocytoid-type cells are not always represented, whereas plasmacytoid and lymphoplasmacytic differentiation is frequently observed [30, 37]. In our case, histology confirmed a lymphoma made up of small diffuse tumour lymphocytes, completely obliterating the lymph node architecture, with marked nuclear atypia. Histological criteria help to formulate initial hypotheses, but are not sufficient to make a definitive diagnosis. They guide the immunohistochemical study, which should be as broad as possible.IHC is essential and therefore requires other small B-cell lymphomas to be ruled out in the diagnosis. Our case had been immunostained using anti:CD20 antibodies (intense and diffuse positive staining of the cytoplasm of the tumour cells); Bcl2 (medium intensity and diffuse nuclear and cytoplasmic labelling of the cytoplasm and nuclear membrane affecting 50% of tumour cells); CD5 (no labelling of tumour cells); CD3 (no labelling of tumour cells); Bcl1 or Cyclin D1 (no labelling of tumour cells); CD10 (no labelling of tumour cells); CD23 (no labelling of tumour cells); Ki67 (high intensity nuclear labelling affecting around 30% of tumour cells). Antibodies to CD5, CD3, Bcl1, CD10 and CD23 are exclusion markers. In the literature, lymphoma cells have a B phenotype: CD20 positive, CD79a positive, PAX5 positive, IgD negative, with CD43 frequently expressed, while CD5 expression is much rarer in 15% of cases. CD23 is generally negative and is only seen in 1/3 of cases. Cyclin D1 (Bcl1) is negative and CG markers (CD10, Bcl6, HGAL, MEF2B) are not observed. Bcl2 is most often positive [4, 38, 41]. These data corroborate our immunohistochemical results, with the exception of certain markers which were not available. The clinical, paraclinical, histological and immunohistochemical data led to the conclusion of a localised lymph node marginal zone lymphoma with a large tumour mass according to the GELF criteria [48, 51].

Asymptomatic patients with no tumour syndrome criteria, as defined by GELF, are followed up regularly without treatment [49].

In symptomatic patients requiring treatment, the therapeutic approach will differ depending on whether the disease is localised or more systemic. For localised disease, surgery followed by radiotherapy is a possible option. Symptomatic patients with no tumour syndrome criteria may also benefit from chlorambucil-based monochemotherapy, ideally combined with rituximab [49].

Patients with one of the GELF criteria should receive rituximab-based immunochemotherapy, such as "R-CVP" (rituximab, cyclophosphamide, vincristine and prednisone), possibly combined with an anthracycline "R-CHOP" (Rituximab - Cyclophosphamide - Hydroxy Doxorubicin Vincristine Prednisone).

Bendamustine in combination with rituximab is indicated in the presence of poor prognostic factors [49]. Our patient therefore benefited from chemotherapy to reduce tumour mass using a combination of cyclophosphamide, vincristine sulphate, doxorubicin hydrochloride (Adriamycin methotrexate), cytarabine and the steroid hormone dexamethasone (Hyper-CVAD) while awaiting the institution of a specific chemotherapy protocol for marginal zone lymphoma. The treatment was a success, melting all the cervical lymph nodes and completely eliminating the pain. The patient's general condition remains well preserved.The specific treatment phase is underway using the Rituximab- CHOP (R-CHOP) protocol. The patient will receive six (06) courses of R-CHOP (one course every 21 days) followed by Rituximab every 2 months for 2 years. In rare cases, antiviral treatment can be effective in patients infected with the hepatitis C virus [49]. Regardless of the treatment used (observation alone, surgical resection, chemotherapy, radiotherapy, steroids), overall survival over 5 years is 60 to 70% [4, 49].

CONCLUSION

Ganglion marginal zone lymphoma is a relatively rare small-cell B lymphoma. The heterogeneity of the histological presentation and the absence of specific immunohistochemical or molecular markers make its diagnosis difficult. Although it is characterised by a very different clinical presentation from MZSL and MALT-type lymphoma, striking similarities in their epidemiology and tumour cell biology confirm a common origin in marginal zone B cells, making clinical findings very difficult. LZMG is diagnosed only after other indolent B-cell lymphoproliferative disorders have been ruled out. The prognosis for MGZL is very encouraging, but aggressive transformation can occur, hence the need for in-depth research to structure recommendations for diagnosis, evaluation and management.

At the end of this work, we put forward some suggestions and recommendations to contribute to the management of patients with lymph node marginal zone lymphoma.

❖ **To the Minister of Health and Public Hygiene**

- Equipping the pathological anatomy and cytology laboratory at the Fada N'gourma Regional Hospital with standard histology equipment.
- Promote universal health insurance to enable lymphoma patients to benefit from systematic histological and immunohistochemical studies.
- Pooling resources with the histo-embryology and cytogenetics department and private facilities in Burkina Faso with molecular biology and cytogenetics laboratories (Hôpital Saint Camille, CERBA) so that lymphoma patients can benefit from molecular and cytogenetic analysis.

❖ **Attending physicians**

Any lymph node swelling suspected of being malignant should be referred for anatomopathological examination as soon as possible.

❖ **To the Head of the Morphology and Organogenesis Laboratory of the Doctoral School of Science and Health of the Joseph KI-ZERBO University of Ouagadougou**

Enhance the panel of antibodies already available, so that pathologists can carry out a more complete immunohistochemical study.

❖ **Medical pathologists**

Create a digital platform dedicated to distance continuing education in order to update knowledge while reducing the need for doctors to travel away from their place of work.

REFERENCES

1. Bontoux C, Bruneau J, Molina TJ. Pathological classification of chronic B lymphoproliferative disorders. Presse médicale. 2019 ; 48(7- 8) :792-806.

2. International Agency for Research on Cancer. World Health Organization: Cancer Today/ Population Fact Sheets, GLOBOCAN 2020, available at http://globocan.iarc.fr/Pages/fact_sheets_population.aspx consulted on 12/01/2024.

3. Christophe B, Marie L, Catherine VK et al. Current management of marginal zone lymphoma, Rev Med Suisse 2015; 11: 1549-56.

4. Swerdlow SH, Campo E, Harris NL, et al. WHO classification of tumours of haematopoietic and lymphoid tissues (Revised 4th edition). Lyon: IARC; 2017.

5. Zucca E, Bertoni F. The spectrum of MALT lymphoma at different sites: biological and therapeutic relevance. Blood. 2016;127:2082-2092.

6. De Wolf-Peeters C, Delabie J. Anatomy and histophysiology of lymphoid tissue. Semin. Oncol 1993;20(6):555-569.

7. Dr Djaalab M. Histology of lymphoid organs and tissues. Histologie spéciale 2ème année médecine. Accessed at https://fac.umc.edu.dz/vet/Cours_Ligne/cours_21_22/Histologie_A2/TP_hist ologie_org_%20lymph.pdf, on 18 January 2024.

8. Histology and embryology laboratory. Lymph nodes. UFR de medecine de Nantes. Visited at https://histologie.univ- nantes.fr/?p=768, on 18January 2024.

9. Fugmann SD, Lee AI, Shockett PE, Villey IJ, Schatz DG The RAG proteins and V(D)J recombination: complexes, ends, and transposition. Annu Rev Immunol. 2000 ; 18 : 495-527.

10. McHeyzer-Williams LJ, Malherbe LP, McHeyzer-Williams MG. Checkpoints in memory B-cell evolution. Immunol Rev. 2006 Jun ; 211 : 255-68.

11. Weill JC., Weller S., Reynaud CA. Human marginal zone B cells. Annu Rev Immunol. 2009 ; 27 :267-85.

12. Vinuesa CG, Tangye SG, Moser B, Mackay CR. Follicular B helper T cells in antibody responses and auto immunity. Nat Rev Immunol. 2005 Nov ; 5(11) :853-65.

13. Lanzavecchia A., Bernasconi N., Traggiai E., Ruprecht CR., Corti D., Sallusto F. Understanding and making use of human memory B cells. Immunol Rev. 2006 Jun ; 211 : 303-9.

14. Maes B., De Wolf-Peeters C. Marginal zone cell lymphoma--an update on recent advances. Histopathology. 2002; 40: 117-126.

15. Harris NL, Jaffe ES, Stein H, et al. A revised European-American Classification of lymphoid neoplasms. A proposal from the International Lymphoma Study Group. Blood. 1994 ; 84 : 1361-1392.

16. Mebius RE., Kraal G. Structure and function of the spleen. Nat rev Immunol, 2005 ; 5 : 606-16.

17. Algara P., Mateo MS., Sanchez-Beato M., et al. Analysis of the IgV(H) somatic mutations in splenic marginal zone lymphoma defines a group of unmutated cases with frequent 7q deletion and adverse clinical course. Blood. 2002 ; 99 : 1299-1304.

18. Farinha P., Gascoyne R. Helicobacter pylori and MALT Lymphoma. Gastroenterology. 2005; 128: 1579-1605.

19. Suarez F., Lortholary O., Hermine O., Lecuit M. Infection-associated lymphomas derived from marginal zone B cells: a model of antigen-driven lymphoproliferation. Blood. 2006 ; 107 : 3034-3044.

20. . Hermine O., Lefrere F., Bronowicki J., et al. Regression of splenic lymphoma with villous lymphocytes after treatment of hepatitis C virus infection. N. Engl J. Med. 2002; 11: 89-94.

21. Khalil MO, Morton LM, Devesa SS, et al. Incidence of marginal zone

lymphoma in the United States, 2001-2009 with a focus on primary anatomic site. Br J Haematol 2014;165:67-77.

22. Gitelson E, Al-Saleem T, Robu V, Millenson MM, Smith MR. Pediatric nodal marginal zone lymphoma may develop in the adult population. Leuk Lymphoma 2010;51(1):89e94.

23. Aqil B, Merritt BY, Elghetany MT, Kamdar KY, Lu XY, Curry CV. Childhood nodal marginal zone lymphoma with unusual clinicopathologic and cytogenetic features for the pediatric variant: a case report. Pediatr Dev Pathol 2015;18(2):167e71.

24. Taddesse-Heath L, Pittaluga S, Sorbara L, Bussey M, Raffeld M, Jaffe ES. Marginal zone B-cell lymphoma in children and young adults. Am J Surg Pathol 2003;27:522-31.

25. O'Suoji C, Welch JJ, Perkins SL, et al. Rare pediatric non-Hodgkin lymphomas: a report from Children's oncology group study ANHL 04B1. Pediatr Blood Cancer 2016;63(5):794e800.

26. Sheibani K, Sohn CC, Burke JS [et al]. Monocytoid B-cell lymphoma. A novel B-cell neoplasm. The American journal of pathology 1986 Aug; 124(2): 310- 318.

27. Cousar JB, McGinn DL, Glick AD [et al]. Report of an unusual lymphoma arising from parafollicular B-lymphocytes (PBLs) or so-called "monocytoid" lymphocytes. Am J Clin Pathol 1987 Jan; 87(1): 121-128.

28. Piris MA, Rivas C, Morente M [et al.]. Monocytoid B-cell lymphoma, a tumour related to the marginal zone. Histopathology 1988 Apr; 12(4): 383-392.

29. Isaacson PGN, B.N.; Piris, M.A.; Berger, F.; Harris, N.L.; Müller-Hermelink, H.K; Swerdlow, S. Nodal marginal zone B-cell lymphoma. In: Jaffe ES, H.; Vardiman, JW. (ed). Pathology and Genetics of Tumors of Haematopoietic and Lymphoid Tissues. Lyon: IARC Press; 2001, pp 161.

30. Campo EP, SA; Jaffe, ES; Müller-Hermelink, HK; Nathwani, BN. Nodal marginal zone lymphoma. In: Swerdlow SH, NL; Jaffe, ES; Pileri, SA; Stein, H;

Jurgen, T; Vardiman, JW. (ed). WHO Classification of Tumours of

Haematopoietic and Lymphoid Tissues. Lyon: IARC Press; 2008, pp 218-219.

31. Boveri E, Arcaini L, Merli M [et al.]. Bone marrow histology in marginal

zone B-cell lymphomas: correlation with clinical parameters and flow cytometry

in 120 patients. Annals of oncology : official journal of the European Society for

Medical Oncology / ESMO 2009 Jan; 20(1): 129-136.

32. Traverse-Glehen A, Bertoni F, Thieblemont C et al. Nodal marginal zone B-

cell lymphoma: a diagnostic and therapeutic dilemma. Oncology (Williston

Park, NY) 2012 Jan; 26(1): 92-99, 103-104.

33. Arcaini L, Lucioni M, Boveri E [et al.]. Nodal marginal zone lymphoma:

current knowledge and future directions of an heterogeneous disease. Eur J

Haematol 2009 Sep; 83(3): 165-174.

34. Ifrah Norbert, Cahn Jean-Yves. Haematology 2nd edition SFH référentiel

des collèges. Masson 2014 : 358p .

35. Iyer VK. Pediatric Lymphoma Diagnosis: Role of FNAC, Biopsy,

Immunohistochemistry and Molecular Diagnostics. Indian J Pediatr.2013 Sep ;

80(9):756-763.

36. Lai C, Roschewski M. Nodal marginal zone lymphoma: impersonalized

medicine. Oncology 2012;26:33-43.

37. Camacho FI, Algara P, Mollejo M, et al. Nodal marginal zone lymphoma: a

heterogeneous tumor: a comprehensive analysis of a series of 27 cases. Am J

Surg Pathol 2003;27:762-71.

38. Mohamed E, Izidore S, Roger A, Yasodha N. Immunoarchitectural Patterns

in Nodal Marginal Zone B-Cell Lymphoma. A Study of 51 Cases. Am J Clin

Pathol 2009;132:39-49.

39. Traverse-Glehen A, Felman P, Callet-Bauchu E, et al. A clinicopathological

study of nodal marginal zone B-cell lymphoma: a report on 21 cases.

Histopathology. 2006;48:162-173.

40. Anamarija M. Lymphoma of the ganglionic marginal zone. Visited on

https://www-pathologyoutlines-com.translate.goog/topic/lymphomanodalMZL.html?_x_tr_sl=en&_x_tr_tl=fr&_x_tr_hl=en&_x_tr_pto=sc, 21 January 2024.

41. SpinaV. et al. Molecular pathogenesis of splenic and nodal marginal zone lymphoma Best Pract Res Clin Haematol (2017).

42. Callet-Bauchu E, Baseggio L, Felman P, Traverse-Glehen A, et al,. Cytogenetic analysis delineates a spectrum of chromosomal changes that can distinguish non-MALT marginal zone B-cell lymphomas among mature B-cell entities: a description of 103 cases. Leukemia. 2005;19:1818-23.

43. Alexandra T, Camille L, Lucile B. Morphological diagnosis of splenic and lymph node marginal zone lymphomas. Horizons Hémato. July-August-September 2019. Volume 09, Issue 03.

44. ZuccaE, ConconiA, LaszloD, . Addition of rituximab to chlorambucil produces superior event-free survival in the treatment of patients with extranodal marginal-zone B-cell lymphoma: 5-year analysis of the IELSG-19 randomized study. J Clin Oncol 2013;31:565-72.

45. RummelMJ, NiederleN, MaschmeyerG, . Bendamustine plus rituximab versus CHOP plus rituximab as first-line treatment for patients with indolent and mantle-cell lymphomas: An open-label, multicentre, randomised, phase 3 non-inferiority trial. Lancet 2013 ;381 :1203-10.

46. FedericoM, LuminariS, DondiA, . R-CVP versus R-CHOP versus R-FM for the initial treatment of patients with advanced-stage follicular lymphoma: Results of the FOLL05 trial conducted by the Fondazione Italiana Linfomi. J Clin Oncol 2013;31:1506-13.

47. Kahl B, Yang D. Marginal zone lymphomas: management of nodal, splenic, and MALT NHL. Hematology Am Soc Hematol Educ Program. 2008;359-364.

48. National Cancer Institute. Adult Non-Hodgkin LymphomaTreatment (PDQ®) Health Professional Version.2015: http://www.cancer.gov/types/lymphoma/hp/adult-nhl-treatment- pdq#section/all,

visited on 21 January 2024.

49. Christophe B, Marie L, Catherine VK, Yves B, Dominique B. Current management of marginal zone lymphoma.Swiss Medical Journal. August 2015, visited on the website https://www.revmed.ch/revue-medicale-suisse/2015/swiss-medical-journal-483/actual-treatment-of-lymphoma-of-the-marginal-zone#tab5, 23 January 2024.

50. Luca A, Marco L, Emanuela B, Marco P. Nodal marginal zone lymphoma: current knowledge and future directions of an heterogeneous disease . European journal of haematology. 2009 September ;83(3) :165-74.

51. Solal-CelignyP, RoyP, ColombatP, . Follicular lymphoma international prognostic index. Blood 2004; 104:1258-65.

52. Dilip Sandipan Nikam. A case report of nodal marginal zone lymphoma: Diagnosis and management. Asian Journal of Oncology 2017 ;Vol3 ; 78-80.

53. Sung Y, Baek-YR , Won S et all . Nodal marginal zone B-cell lymphoma: analysis of 36 cases. Clinical presentation and treatment outcomes of nodal marginal zone B-cell lymphoma. Ann Hematol (2006) 85:781-786 .

54. Frampas E. Lymphomas: some basics the radiologist needs to know. Journal of Diagnostic and Interventional Radiology (2013) 94, 135-149.

SUMMARY

***Title** : Lymphoma of the ganglion marginal zone: about a case diagnosed at the regional hospital of Fada N'Gourma.*

***Introduction**: Marginal zone lymphomas (MZL) are subdivided into three entities: extraganglionic MZL developed from mucosa-associated lymphoid tissue (MALT), splenic MZL (SZML) and lymph node MZL (GNML). MGL is a relatively rare small-cell B-cell lymphoma. We report the case of a 52-year-old patient with MGL diagnosed at the Fada N'Gourma Regional Hospital.*

***Case report**: A 52-year-old patient with a history of chronic viral hepatitis B presented with a painful left cervical mass. Symptoms began 9 months ago with the appearance of a painful, progressive left cervical mass. Clinical examination revealed multiple painful left laterocervical adenopathies. Blood tests showed an increase in lacticodehydrogenase (391.3 IU/L) and beta-2-microglobulin (2.92 mg/L). A cervico-thoraco-abdomino-pelvic CT scan showed four (04) left latero-cervical adenomegalia measuring 18mm, 15mm, 14mm and 9mm. Histology of the lymph node excisions revealed diffuse tumour proliferation. The tumour cells were small, with sparse eosinophilic cytoplasm and irregular, hyperchromatic and often nucleolated nuclei. Nuclear atypia was marked and mitotic figures rare. Immunohistochemistry showed intense, diffuse cytoplasmic labelling of tumour cells with anti-CD20 antibody; moderate-intensity, diffuse cytoplasmic and nuclear labelling of approximately 50% of tumour cells with anti-Bcl2 antibody. Ki67 was intensely expressed by 30% of tumour lymphocytes. The diagnosis was localized lymphoma of the lymph node marginal zone with a large tumour mass.*

***Conclusion**: Ganglion marginal zone lymphoma is a relatively rare small cell B-cell lymphoma. The heterogeneity of the histological presentation and the absence of specific immunohistochemical or molecular markers make its* *diagnosis difficult.*

Key words *: Lymphoma, lymph node marginal zone, histology, immunohistochemistry, Fada N'Gourma.*

Author*: PITROIPA Judith Gueswendé, judith_pitroipa@yahoo.fr, Tel ; 70103194.*

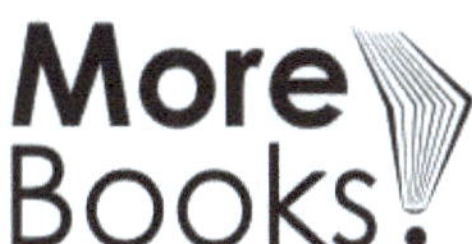

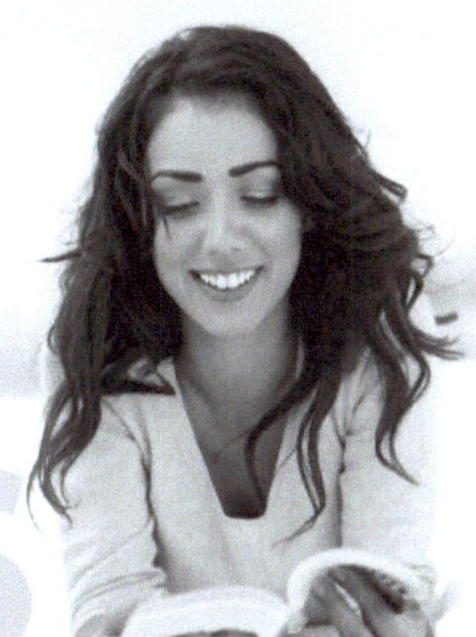

I want morebooks!

Buy your books fast and straightforward online - at one of world's fastest growing online book stores! Environmentally sound due to Print-on-Demand technologies.

Buy your books online at
www.morebooks.shop

Kaufen Sie Ihre Bücher schnell und unkompliziert online – auf einer der am schnellsten wachsenden Buchhandelsplattformen weltweit! Dank Print-On-Demand umwelt- und ressourcenschonend produziert.

Bücher schneller online kaufen
www.morebooks.shop

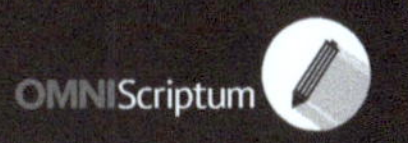

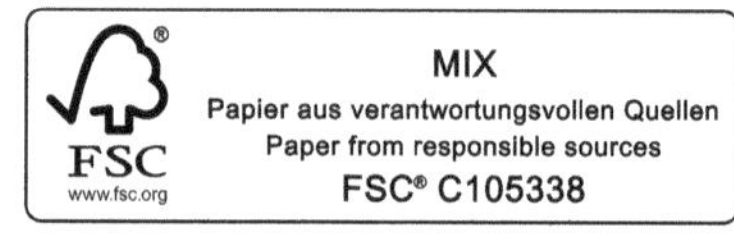

Printed by Books on Demand GmbH, Norderstedt / Germany